You Were Smaller Than a Dot

Glen C. Griffin, M.D.

Illustrated by Carol Jeanne Ehlers
Cover by Sherry Thompson

Deseret Book Company
Salt Lake City, Utah
1980

© 1980 Glen C. Griffin
All rights reserved
Printed in the United States of America
ISBN 0-87747-817-1
Library of Congress Catalog No. 72-90685

A Few Words for Parents

You Were Smaller Than a Dot was written in response to hundreds of requests from parents who have been looking for a simple children's book to help introduce the wonderful story of how human life begins.

Certainly a child can learn something about sex from the kid down the street, or from lots of other sources. But what is learned? Maybe some very real facts, but probably some things that are not quite right, too. When it comes to teaching children about sex, a parent might ask, "If not me, who?" "If not now, when?" Children want answers when they think up questions. Being put off encourages them to seek information elsewhere. But if a parent captures teaching moments as they come along, messages about self-worth, values, and families can be given along with physical facts. *You Were Smaller Than a Dot* is a beginning.

When should more be said? Whenever more is asked, or at least every year or so in one-to-one parent-child chats. Several levels of explanation could be given about how an engine works—one that will correctly answer a five-year-old's question, another an eight-year-old's, and still another that of a student in auto mechanics. Even then, the whole course is not given in one lesson.

"How does the sperm get inside the mother?" asked by a little child might be answered by "The father puts it there." Later a more specific explanation is indicated. Two other books for older children, *About You . . . and Other Important People* and *Not About Birds,* have been written by the author and his wife, Mary Ella Griffin, R.N.

Truthful answers are really rather simple. As a parent listens and answers direct and indirect questions, a relationship of open communication begins to grow. By the way, you too were smaller than a dot!

Foreword

You Were Smaller Than a Dot should be in every home where there are children. This little primer presents appropriate answers to questions all children either ask or wonder about. What a help it can be for parents!

This attractive book was carefully created to provide an optimum teaching experience for those of young and curious ages. The author, Dr. Glen C. Griffin, is a well-known pediatrician and writer. His articles about children and teens have helped thousands of parents.

Your children will love *You Were Smaller Than a Dot*. I recommend it highly.

James B. Gillespie, M.D.
Past President
American Academy of Pediatrics

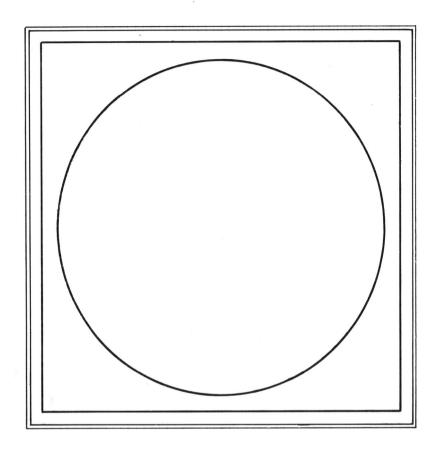

Can you find a baby picture
to paste here?

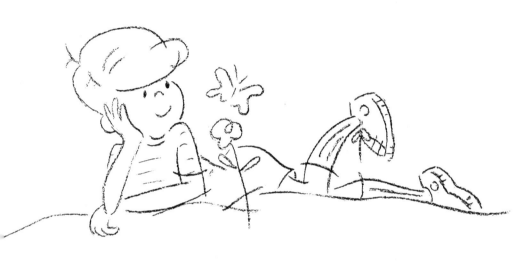

This is a story about *you,*
a story that began years ago . . .

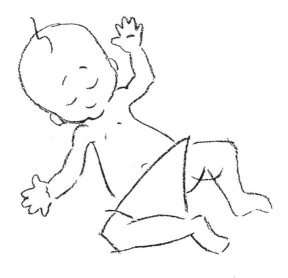

even before you were a little baby.

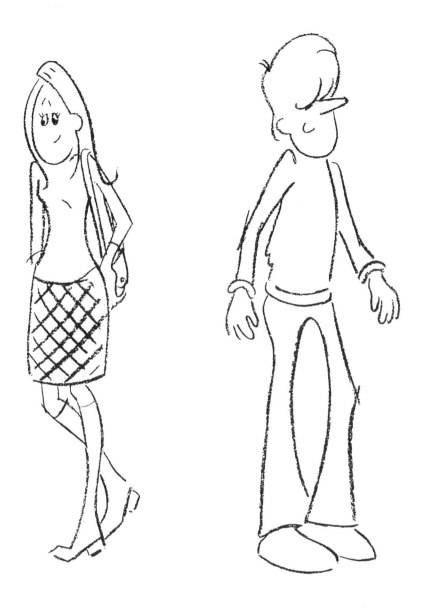

A long time ago your mother
and father didn't even know
each other.

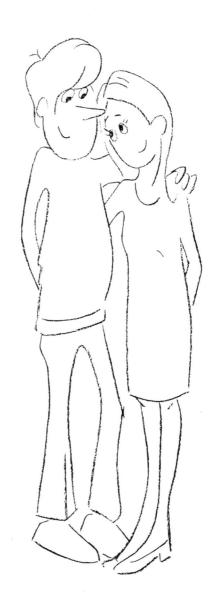

Then they met, fell in love,

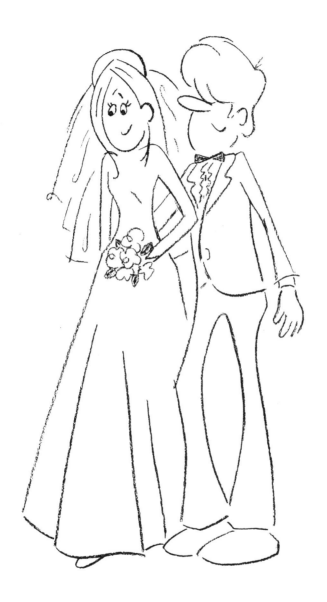

and decided to get married.

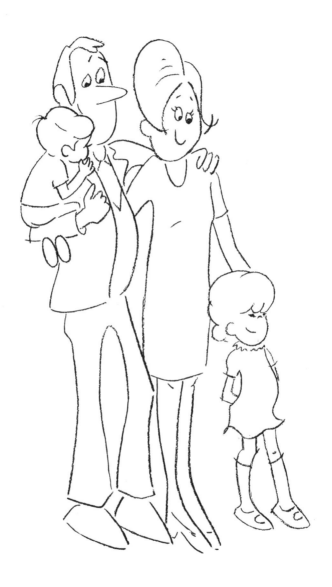

Since a family is happier
with children,

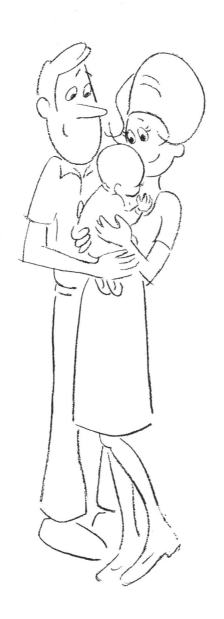

your mother and father
wanted a baby.

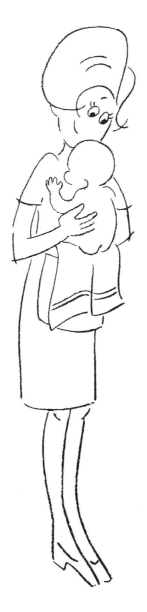

They wanted *you* . . .
to love and to care for.

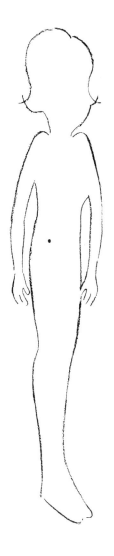

This is how it all happens.
A baby begins as a tiny egg,
inside a mother.

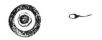

Then this little egg is joined
by a small sperm from the father
so it can grow into a baby.

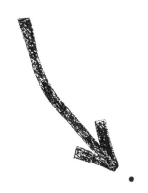

Both the sperm and the egg together
are even smaller than a dot—
and that's how small *you* once were!

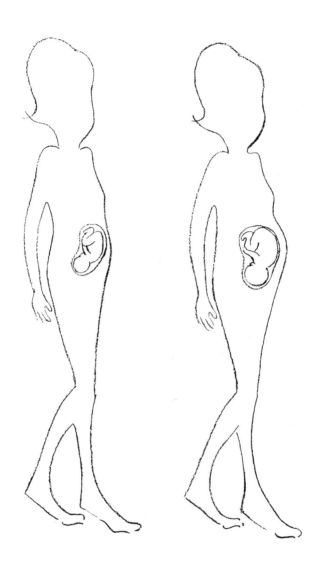

Then this little dot grows into a baby
in a safe, warm place (the uterus)
inside the mother.

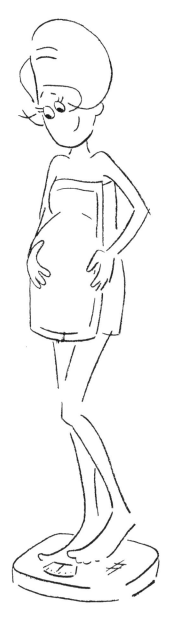

The baby grows bigger and bigger . . .
the uterus grows bigger and bigger . . .
and so does the mother!

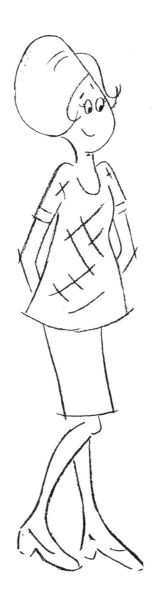

When a baby is growing in the
uterus, the mother is pregnant.

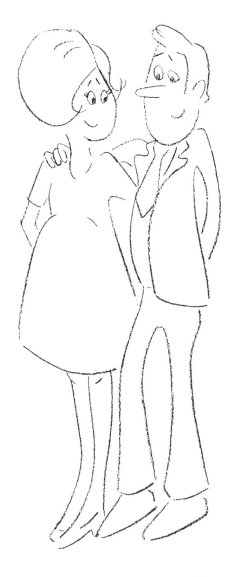

This is a happy time for parents
as they think about their baby
who will soon be born.

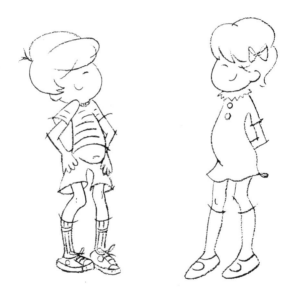

Before *you* were born, your mother
and father thought and thought
about you . . . wondering if you
would be a boy or a girl . . .

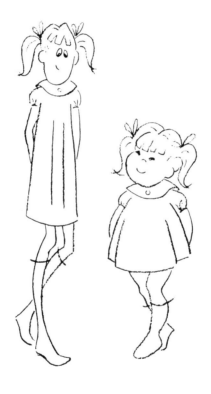

what color eyes you would have . . .
if you would be little or big . . .
and many other things about you.

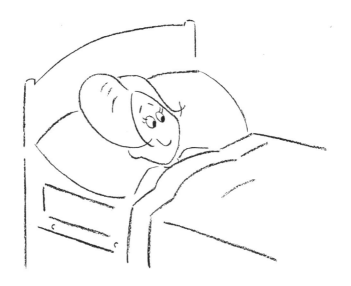

When a baby is ready to be born,
the mother may go to a hospital,
where doctors and nurses take
care of her.

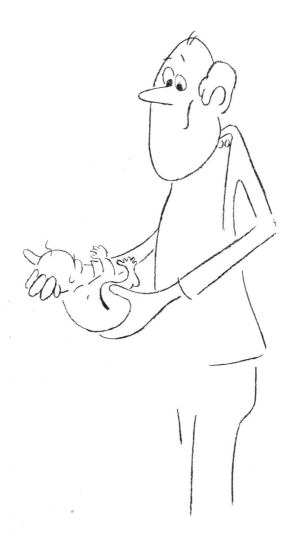

The baby comes out of the mother's
uterus and out of the mother through
an opening called the vagina.

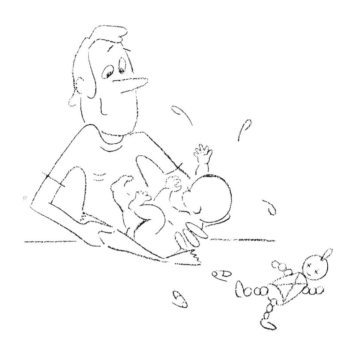

You were a special baby,
even though you cried quite a bit . .
needed your diaper changed . . .

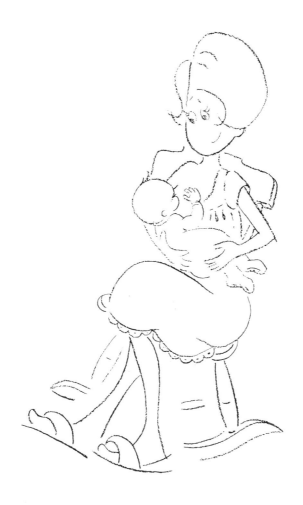

and had to be fed every little while,
either from mother's breasts or
from a baby bottle.

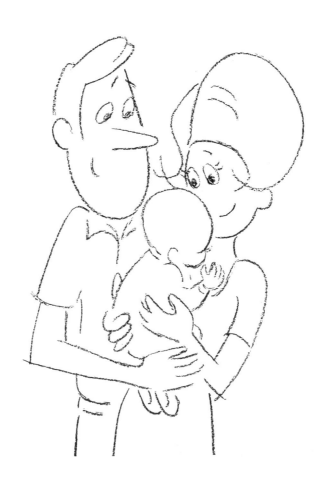

Your being born made your
mother and father very happy.
They love you, and they always will

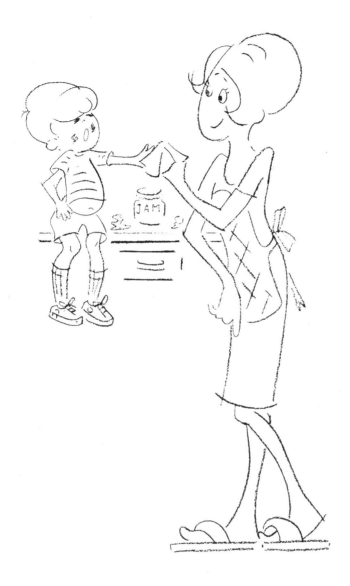

They like being with you . . .
and they like to hear you talk and
ask questions.

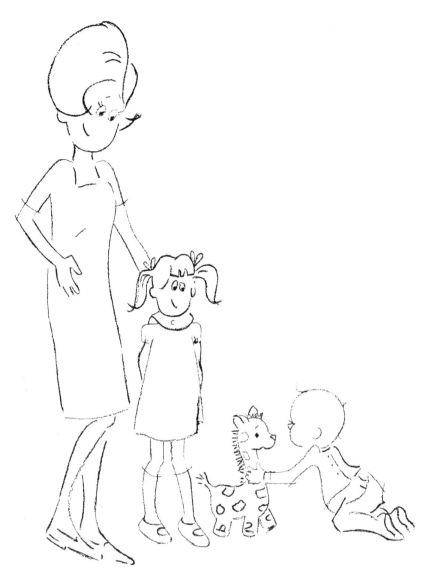

As the years go by and you grow up,
you will probably get married
and have children of your own to
teach and to love. And someday *you*
may read this little book to *them*!

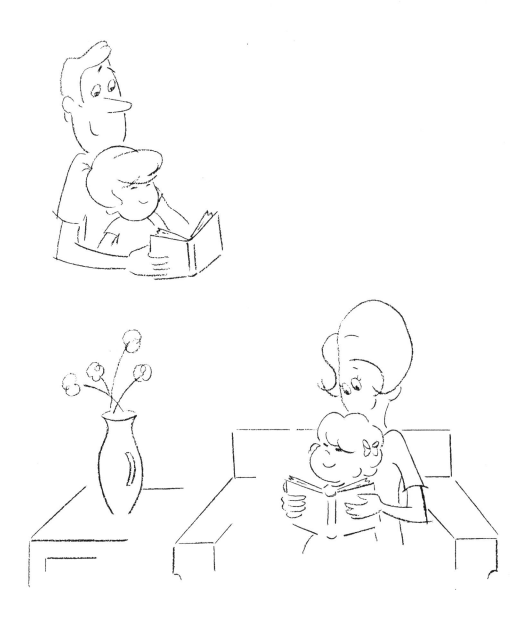

So ask them to tell you more
about when you were a baby
and about other things you
want to know.